I0439417

TABLE OF CONTENTS

Drop Three Dress Sizes in 30-Days
Beyond Dieting
©2012 Dr. Harry Jay

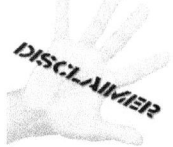

DISCLAIMER AND TERMS OF USE AGREEMENT:

(Please Read This Before Using This Book)

This information is for educational and informational purposes only. The content is not intended to be a substitute for any professional advice, diagnosis, or treatment.

The authors and publisher of this book and the accompanying materials have used their best efforts in preparing this book.

The authors and publisher make no representation or warranties with respect to the accuracy, applicability, fitness, or completeness of the contents of this book. The information contained in this book is strictly for educational purposes. Therefore, if you wish to apply ideas contained in this book, you are taking full responsibility for your actions.

The authors and publisher disclaim any warranties (express or implied), merchantability, or fitness for any particular purpose. The author and publisher shall in no event be held liable to any party for any direct, indirect, punitive, special, incidental or other consequential damages arising directly or indirectly from any use of this material, which is provided "as is", and without warranties. As always, the advice of a competent legal, tax, accounting, medical or other professional should be sought where applicable.

The authors and publisher do not warrant the performance, effectiveness or applicability of any sites listed or linked to in this book. All links are for information purposes only and are not warranted for content, accuracy or any other implied or explicit purpose. No part of this may be copied, or changed in any format, or used in any way other than what is outlined within this course under any circumstances. Violators will be prosecuted.

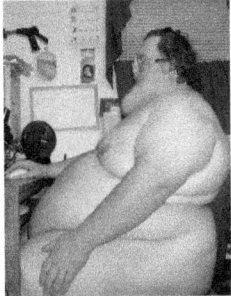

No way...yes WAY!

The picture above is downright frightening. But you only have to watch some reality show on TV to see just how devastating some people have become with their so-called reliance on food.

Chances are none of my readers are this far gone but the causes of severe obesity are the same as moderate obesity.

This book is not for wussie people that expect a pill or a dieting program that removes weight just by thinking about it. It is not about blab it and grab it, dream it and be it, say it and claim it or any of the other nonsense that we all see published seemingly everywhere.

This book is about sound behavioral science and getting you to learn and understand that your mind controls everything! But the first think you need to learn and understand is what we call in science "FIRST CAUSE"!

Question #1: Is someone who is addicted to cocaine a cocaine addict because they ingest cocaine?

Question #2: A person who tells a lie is a liar because he/she tells a lie?

In both cases, the manifested behavior – ingestion of cocaine and telling a lie – is the result of some underlying problem or issue that causes a person to self medicate themselves away from the stress and anxiety as in the case of cocaine addiction or is the result of some internal fantasy that has become a belief system as in the case of the liar.

In other words, many people confuse the manifested behavior as the cause and in the case of overeating, this is very much true.

Overeating is not the problem; overeating is the effect of the cause and the cause can be boredom, low self esteem, loneliness, depression, and tons more.

So we will delve deep into First Cause as I go along and remember to keep things in perspective.

Okay, the art of being fit includes adopting and maintaining an optimum weight level that matches your body needs and level of activity. There are various fitness and wellness agencies that publish weight charts but I wouldn't be too eager to go in search of them since most of them are dead wrong.

Dieting involves two things:
1. Physical reduction of calories and/or the increase in activity
2. Using the power of the mind to reduce your weight

In this book, I will be discussing both ways. Food can be and most often is an addiction. The Federal Government defines a drug as "anything that alters the physiological structure of the body," which according to them, food is a drug!

The art of controlling yourself in anything you do begins in the mind and dieting and optimum weight level is no exception.

In my book, "The Denial of Self" http://www.amazon.com/dp/B008B7OK32, I define the core essential to all if not most of our problems – gratification of SELF!

Now stop for just a moment and think about your life and the problems you have caused by the need to seek self gratification. I think you will be totally amazed to find that most if not all of your problems stem from this need. But it doesn't have to be this way! By learning how to control your mind, you can literally control your whole life and not just your weight.

And remember, self gratification is the "effect" of some underlying "cause"!!!

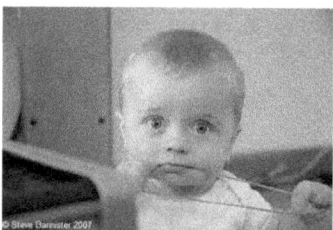

Assuming that there is no physical or nutritional malady affecting your weight (such as Toxemia), maintaining an optimum weight level is more mental than it is physical.

In fact, anything and everything you do is more mental than physical since the mind controls all behavior/action/conduct.

What I mean by this is simple: most people can and will be successful in weight loss; however, without controlling the initial "First Cause" of weight gain, chances are you will gain all the weight back again.

I have written extensively in the past on how many diet programs fail because they do not change the person's subconscious mind habits and personal food choices that the person held prior to dieting.

Once the person has finished dieting, he/she returns to his/her old habits and practices and once again begins to gain weight. It is called "The Vicious Circle of Weight Gain".

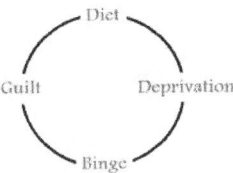

Example: A 36 year old lady had a habit of eating at night prior to bedtime. Once she stopped this habit; her optimum body weight returned. Eating at night also caused this lady insomnia, which also went away.

But guess what?

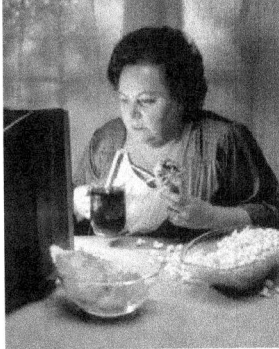

She went back to her old habits and gained the weight back and also the insomnia even after experiencing how much better she felt. The reason she did this is because she never addresses the mind problem of the subconscious First Cause for eating at night.

Pardon the pun but I won't leave you in the dark. It turns out after a few counseling sessions that the reason for her eating at night was that she was afraid of the night and she ate to keep herself awake.

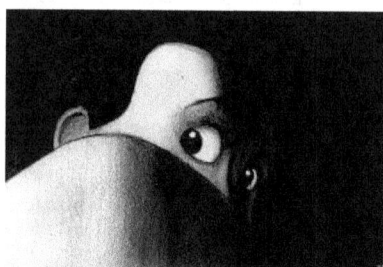

There are a plethora of diet programs available on the net today; most of which ignore the mental aspects of dieting.

Statistics show that the American population is increasing in weight; but nowhere in these statistics does it allow for any of the many mental reasons for gaining weight; only the physical reasons such as lack of exercise, overeating, sedentary lifestyle etc.

The way you lose weight and the efficiency of any diet is determined by habits, exercise, age, gender, and more and we will address these issues too.

I offer two websites that are synergistic to what I will be teaching you and that can provide more information:

http://healthfitnesswellnessnation.com/
http://appliedmindsciences.com/

I will address in this book both aspects of dieting; the mental as well as physical. I will also show you how to reprogram your mind, which in effect will make your goal of losing weight much easier and almost guarantee that the excessive pounds will not return.

I will even offer you a dieting program that I use to keep my weight at an optimum level since I travel extensively and my exercise program is constantly being interrupted.

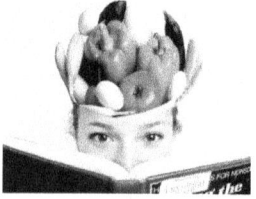

I will begin the true facts about dieting and weight loss then get into the mental aspects of dieting.

I will show you how to reprogram your mind to do anything you desire let alone reprogramming it so that you maintain optimum weight levels.

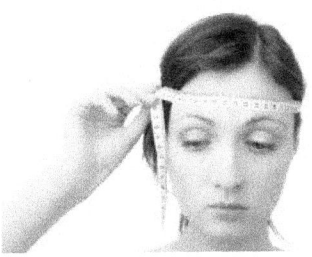

I think you will enjoy the information I give you but as usual; write to me if I can be of assistance harry@epubwealth.com.

Chapter 1 – Truth About Dieting

Although fast weight loss may sound like an appealing idea, it is not wise to do this and from a physiological (the science of the human body) point of view, it is very dangerous. Instead, your physical focus (not mental focus) should be on cutting calories and exercising more to lose weight at a rate of 1 to 2 lbs. weekly! Rapid weight loss actually increases your chances of regaining the lost weight. But, more importantly, it also it puts you at risk for serious medical complications such as.

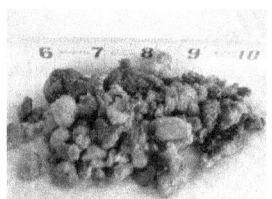

Gallstones - Losing weight at a rate of more than 3 lbs. weekly increases your risk of developing gallstones. Gallstones are small clusters of material that look similar to pebbles and are produced by the gallbladder. They may block the normal flow of bile. Symptoms of gallstones include pain between the shoulder blades and in the upper-right abdomen. You may also have gallstones without experiencing any symptoms. The gallbladder and the liver work together in digestion. The gallbladder produces bile, which allows the liver to aid in digestion of fat…more on this later.

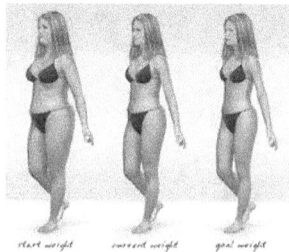

start weight   current weight   goal weight

Weight Gain - You are more likely to regain the weight if you are using a very low-calorie diet or fad diet that is extremely restrictive. You are not likely to be able to follow the plan for a prolonged period of time and once you grow bored with the plan and return to your normal eating patterns, the increased calorie intake will cause you to regain the weight plus more weight. Diets that require fasting periods or involve skipping meals may also cause weight gain as well, because you may compensate at a later time by overeating.

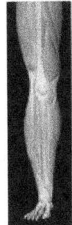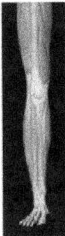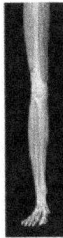

Muscle and Water Loss - The weight that you lose quickly may not actually be fat you are burning; you may be losing water weight or lean muscle tissue. When you are not eating enough calories, muscle tissue may be broken down by the body due to nutritional deficiencies. Certain diets, such as low-carb eating plans, may reduce water retention, and this may be the reason you see the weight come off quickly.

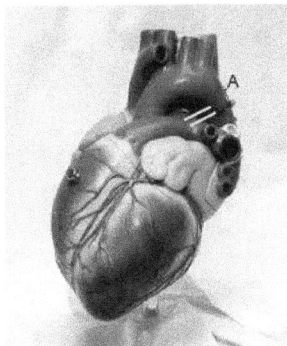

Heart Disorders - Low-calorie diets that require you to consume less than 800 calories per day are particularly dangerous. When you are not eating enough calories, you put yourself at risk for heart irregularities.

A weight loss of 1 to 2 pounds a week is the typical healthy recommendation and although this may sound too slow, it isn't and it is healthy when physical dieting.

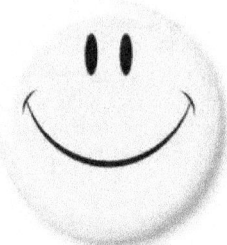

Note: Mental dieting or using the mind to lose weight does not adhere to the recommendation of 1 to 2 pounds per week. By using the mind to reduce weight, the body will lose in varying proportions based on what the mind tells it to do.

Remember that 1 pound (0.45 kilogram) of fat contains 3,500 calories. So to lose 1 pound a week, you need to burn 500 more calories than you eat each day (500 calories x 7 days = 3,500 calories).

Food Choices is the Main Cause of Weight Gain.

- Sugar is your #1 enemy. Stay away from orange juice, bread, artificial sweeteners, cereals, salad dressings, granola, and many health foods that contain high amounts of sugar.

- Processed foods are just as bad and are enemy #2.

- Breads to eat – bread made from sprouted grains, rice, or spelt

- Sweet potatoes, fruits and vegetables are great for fat burning.

- Eating fat does not make you fat; it will actually help you burn fat off your body BUT you have to eat the right kind of fat to do this. Eat the wrong kind of fat and you will STORE FAT.

- Wrong Fats: Avoid hydrogenated oils, canola and vegetable oils, margarine and those substitute fake butter products

- Good Fats: Fats you can eat: real butter, eggs, coconut oil, avocados, nuts, olive oil

- Myth: avoid saturated fats for optimum health…PURE BUPKES!!!

- Sugar is the enemy and not fats! The #1 food source of the body is FAT. The body will frist look for fat to burn before sugars and protein.

Low blood sugar causes food cravings, and fatigue. By eating you increase your blood sugar. If you eat the wrong things like sugar and bad carbs, your blood sugar spikes causing the pancreas to pour insulin into your system. This causes a severe drop in blood sugar and once again the cravings and fatigue occurs and the vicious circle begins again.

Okay, so you have two options to losing weight: physical dieting and by using the power of the mind…but wait!

The mind controls everything you do whether it is eating, sex, working…everything!

In actuality, the success you have with physical dieting will also be controlled by the mind. Your willpower or perseverance is determined by the mind.

So now I am going to teach you about your mind and how to harness it to do anything you want including losing weight.

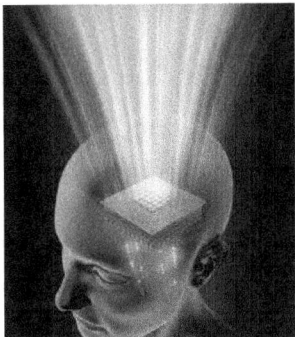

Please don't use this on the dog (lol)!

Chapter 2 – The "Central You" Concept

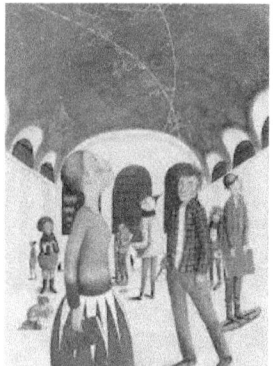

I live in Southern Utah in a big house on many acres of land. My life is real cushy; in the morning I arise very early, take my cup of coffee and go and sit on the patio. All of my senses take in what is happening around me. I can hear the crickets, the air conditioner; I can even hear the water ripple in the pool as the breeze blows. I can watch an owl as it sits patiently for its prey and hear the wildlife in the woods behind my house moving around.

My point in telling you all this is that once I project my senses outward, away from myself, I can see and hear everything.

I am no longer the "center" of my existence. Self is denied!

My mind is not employing any of the filters I have accumulated throughout my life. I am sitting quietly and observing.

Now look at the picture below.

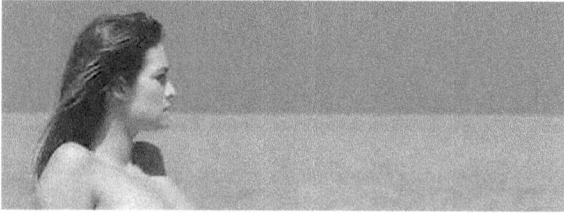

An untrained observer will insert themselves in the picture by telling a story. This story is different between genders as well as maturity but is always a fantasy.

But one essential common element of the story will be that it really has nothing to do with the woman; the story you told yourself is completely about you. Oh, it will involve some type of interaction with the woman but the story will have you at the center.

This is what I call the "Central You" concept.

All sensory input coming into your mind through the five senses are filtered and revolve around you and this includes how you view and analyze weight as you see others around you.

People live their lives with themselves at the center of their universe.

My point is simple: to observe completely you must project your senses away from yourself.

In a study I conducted in 1983, I asked six men ages, 18, 29, 36, 45, 57, and 69 to give me one sentence after they looked at the picture above. Here are their responses

Age 18, "Wow, I hope I meet her some day!"

Age 29: "Although you can see for sure, she is really built."

Age 36: "The picture reminds me of Cancun with my wife."

Age 45: "The woman looks pensive and not relaxed."

Age 57: "Not my type; she looks to me that she is seeking attention."

Age 69: "The first thing that comes to mind is a nudist colony."

Notice that a good majority of the comments were physical in nature. A man's psyche is dominated by the physical and intellectual planes.

We then asked six women to comment on the same picture, ages 17, 24, 33, 41, 52 and 66. Here are their responses:

Age 17: "Nice hair and makeup but she doesn't look happy."

Age 24: "She doesn't seem to care about discretion; she looks topless."

Age 33: "I think she is posing for a picture or something."

Age 41: "She is definitely deep in thought and oblivious to her surroundings."

Age 52: "I certainly hope that isn't a public beach!"

Age 66: "With a figure like that she simply cannot be alone on that beach."

Okay, notice the comments from the women were emotional rather than physical in nature. A woman's psyche is dominated by four planes – emotional, spiritual, physical and intellectual where a man's psyche is dominated by only two – physical and intellectual.

Why is this important? Because weight loss and weight control has different meanings and objectives between genders. Women are more prone to diet because they want to look and feel good, which are both emotional aspects where men primarily want to be fit and trim, which are both physical aspects.

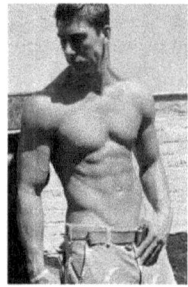
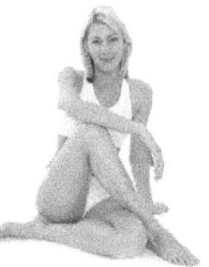

Now look at the picture below.

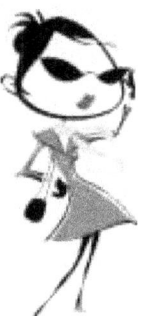

Here is another picture of a woman but this one is not real; it is an animated version. The story you would tell will be different or there would be no story at all. But if there were a story; it would also revolve around you because every fantasy you have is perfect where you are perfect too.

The Mechanism of the Mind

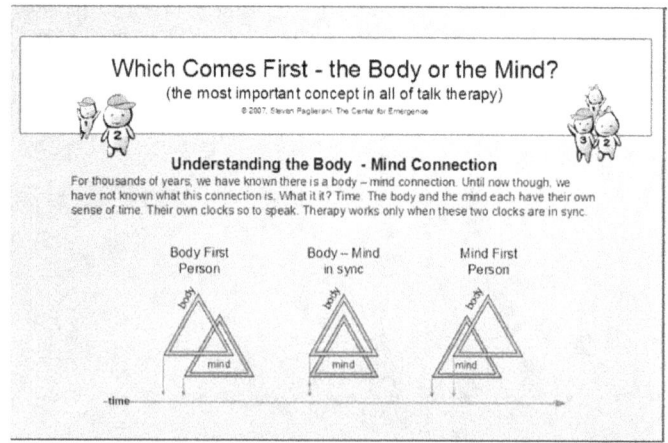

Which Comes First - the Body or the Mind?
(the most important concept in all of talk therapy)
© 2007, Steven Paglierani, The Center for Emergence

Understanding the Body - Mind Connection

For thousands of years, we have known there is a body – mind connection. Until now though, we have not known what this connection is. What it it? Time. The body and the mind each have their own sense of time. Their own clocks so to speak. Therapy works only when these two clocks are in sync.

| Body First Person | Body – Mind in sync | Mind First Person |

Prior to the fall of man into sin as described in the Garden of Eden, man's spirit was hooked to God's infinite spirit. There was no death because God's spirit is infinite. Man is the only animal on earth that shares the eternality nature of God. The subject of eternal life has been a heated topic of man from the beginning of our existence.

In Greek mythology, there's a story about a mortal youth named Tithonus. Aurora, the goddess of dawn, fell in love with the boy and when Zeus, the king of the gods, promised to grant Aurora any gift she chose for her lover, she asked that Tithonus might live forever. But, in her haste she forgot to ask for eternal youth, so when Zeus granted her request, Tithonus was doomed to an eternity of perpetual aging as a grouchy old man... forever.

In the movie "Highlander," Angus McLeod was born in 1518 as an immortal being. He could not die and to me, the best part of the movie was the depiction of this immortal's agony here on earth as he watched everything he loved die forcing him to begin his life over and over again. He saw all of the ugliness, which man had caused over four centuries. He witnessed the Spanish Inquisition, Waterloo, the atrocities of the Third Reich, and more. He saw the slavery and bigotry of the eighteenth century, the slaughter of the Native American tribes after the Civil War. This man's life was a living Hell!

There is a very big difference between the ways our feeble minds picture eternal life versus God's idea of eternal life. Our understanding comes from Quantum Physics and is limited within the Time-Space Continuum.

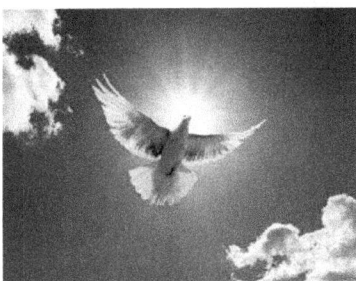

Life is your spirit, but the soul of man has usurped the spirit's position and psychology is now forced to define "how" we live our lives based on the animating force of the soul instead of the spirit. As I said previously, the soul has usurped the spirit's place as our animating force. Let's discuss this now.

- ❖ **Body First Person** - When the body becomes our life, we live as animals.
- ❖ **Body-Mind In Sync** - When the soul becomes our life, we live as rebels and fugitives in a life of desires, emotions, and will (consuming entities). This is the position of mankind today!
- ❖ **Mind First Person** - But when we come to live our life in the mind/spirit and by the spirit, though we still use our soul's faculties just as we do our physical faculties, they are now the servants of the spirit.

If you live as a consuming entity, you will always lose. In other words, to get, you must give - you must sacrifice! Have you ever wondered why you have so many anxieties, phobias, worries and fears? The reality of this world is evil. So what is reality? I will tell you. This is reality:

"Life without war is impossible either in nature or in grace. The basis of physical, mental, moral and spiritual life is antagonism. Health is the balance between physical life and external nature, and it is maintained only by sufficient vitality on the inside against things on the outside. Everything outside my physical life is designed to put me to death. Things, which keep me going when I am alive, disintegrate me when I am dead. If I have enough fighting power, I produce the balance of health. The same is true of mental life. If I want to maintain a vigorous mental life, I have to fight, and in that way the mental balance called thought is produced. Morally it is the same. Everything that does not partake of the nature of virtue is the enemy of virtue in me, and it depends on what moral caliber I have whether I overcome and produce virtue (GOOD CHARACTER). Immediately I fight, I am moral in that particular. No man is virtuous because he cannot help it; virtue (character) is acquired."

- ❖ Psychology only studies the observable aspects of the mind and discounts the unseen or intangible aspects of the human mind.
- ❖ Behavioral science attempts to study the intangible aspects of the human mind…why you do the things you do and more importantly why you don't do what you should do.
- ❖ There is no such thing as commercial psychology versus personal psychology. The mind uses the same mechanism to evaluate all types of relationships.
- ❖ Everything we do revolves around relationships. We relate to our environment, our friends, family, co-workers, other people and even our pets. We are social animals.

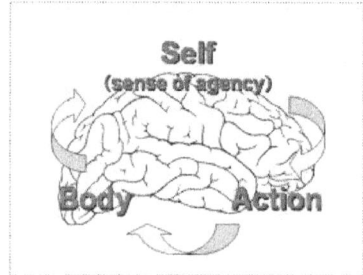

Here is the equation for the Mechanism of the Mind

Belief Systems + Thought + Delight = Action/Behavior/Conduct

Conscious Mind

5-senses:
Sight
Hearing

Taste
Touch
Smell
ESP (women only)

Subconscious Mind

Intellect:
Experiential
Empirical

DEW:
Desires, Emotions and Will

Here is an exercise you might find weird but it demonstrates the power of the human mind.

Fi yuo cna raed tihs, yuo hvae a sgtrane mnid too. Cna yuo raed tihs? Olny 55 plepoe out of 100 can. I cdnuolt blveiee taht I cluod aulaclty uesdnatnrd waht I was rdanieg. The phaonmneal pweor of the hmuan mnid, aoccdrnig to a rscheearch at Cmabrigde Uinervtisy, it dseno't mtaetr in waht oerdr the ltteres in a wrod are, the olny iproamtnt tihng is taht the frsit and lsat ltteer be in the rghit pclae. The rset can be a taotl mses and you can sitll raed it whotuit a pboerlm. Tihs is bcuseae the huamn mnid deos not raed ervey lteter by istlef, but the wrod as a wlohe. Azanmig huh? Yaeh and I awlyas tghuhot slpeling was ipmorantt!

You might have found it somewhat unusual that you could probably read the jumbled mess above. Actually over half the people that see this exercise can decipher the words at the same speed of reading as if the words were not jumbled.

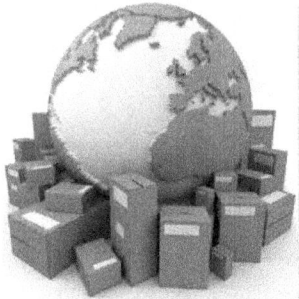

It is important to note that the human mind thinks in packages…concepts rather than individual ideas.

Your eyes see each letter but the mind looks at the whole word instead. As you read, the mind looks at the first and last letter only.

If you were to listen to an orchestra, your ear listens to every note from every instrument but a trained ear can actually pick out individual instruments from the whole sound as the mind hears the whole symphony.

How does this apply to you?

Learning to observe means going beyond the mind's natural ability to only read the first and last letters of a word.

It is training the mind to see all the letters, not just the eye but the mind!

Truisms About the Human Mind

- ❖ Pain vs. Pleasure – people are more motivated to avoid pain than seek pleasure.
- ❖ A person that is suffering depression will seek relief (notice I didn't say cure) before they seek happiness.
- ❖ The human mind cannot tell the difference between fantasy and reality.
- ❖ The human mind gravitates to the desires, emotions and will of its psyche. People grave entertainment so fantasy dominates their existences.
- ❖ The human mind is easily distracted! You can either be the cause of these distractions or other stimuli will be the cause but rest assured people WILL BE distracted because the human mind is gullible.

The human mind responds quickly to these three forms of stimuli

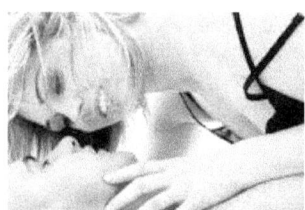 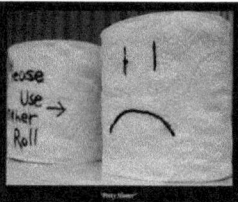 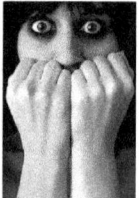

- ❖ Sex
- ❖ Humor
- ❖ FEAR

But the greatest of them all is FEAR!

BTW – on the positive side we have faith, hope, love, but the greatest of these *is* LOVE.

Fear usually takes the form of what is called "Scarcity Thought"

You are afraid that someone will have what you feel belongs to you or that others will have more "stuff" than you.

❖ The subconscious mind is often referred to as the "heart," and is the control mechanism the body uses to store our beliefs.

❖ **These beliefs are stored as pictures in our "hearts" and create frequencies in our bodies.**

❖ We know that the optimum human frequency is a little below 7.83 hertz. To drop below this frequency brings on the onslaught of disease. To rise above it a person demonstrates psychic abilities.

❖ Harmful beliefs that cause unhealthy frequencies are the source of almost all problems - physical, mental, emotional.

❖ The subconscious mind creates a belief system, which we call "pictures of the heart."

❖ These pictures involve either visions, or dreams/fantasies.

❖ Science has discovered that the subconscious mind cannot distinguish between fantasy and reality.

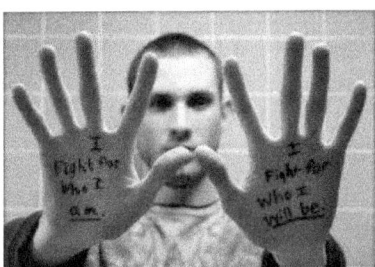

- The subject of all dreams is the dreamer.
- Dreams are born in our desires, emotions and will.
- Dreamers believe in a belief system, which is fantasy.
- A life lived within a fantasy creates a feeling of self-centeredness, hopelessness and despair. In dreams everything is perfect.
- The subject of a vision is not the visionary but the world.
- Visions are born in the intellect.
- Visions are pictures of the future that have already been experienced in the heart of those who give it birth.
- Visionaries sacrifice themselves for the good of mankind.
- Visions have a moral quality that transcends the self-centered nature of dreams.
- By its very nature a vision launches a mission, a "cause-that-inspires."
- Visions create a sense of belonging.

❖ We act upon visions and/or dreams, using thought.

- ❖ Thought employs the intellect, in the case of visions, or the desires, emotions and the will, in the case of dreams.
- ❖ Intellectual thought relies on wisdom; emotional thought relies on the pursuit of pleasure, comfort and delight.
- ❖ Dreamers live within a facade; they create a false sense of worth using imaginary situations.
- ❖ Visionaries live within reality; they create change, within a framework of restraint, and intellectual thought.
- ❖ The world is made up of OPPOSITES, which is usually the corrupted version of the original. We have good and evil. We have love and lust!
- ❖ EVERYTHING YOU DO IS BECAUSE OF LOVE OR LUST. Learn to love because there are no crimes beyond forgiveness.

*Love is born in the intellect; lust is born in the DEW!
*Love is vision; lust is fantasy.
*Love restrains & sacrifices; lust is selfish
*Love is being one with someone or something
*Lust is being with someone or something.
*Visionaries love; dreamers lust!
*Visionaries do what is required; dreamers just do their best!

WHEN THERE IS NO HOPE OF LOVE DO WE ABANDON OURSELVES TO LUST?

Yes we do!

Pictures of the heart are your belief system.

- ❖ We animate these pictures into either fantasies, or visions.
- ❖ People do not appear to see the difference between the matter part of an organism and the life part, which animates it.
- ❖ We seem to think that the organism itself is life. In other words, it is not our outward appearance that is our life, but our inward existence.
- ❖ Life is what goes into the body. Death is what comes out.
- ❖ A person who lies is not a liar because he tells a lie. The lie is the manifested behavior of some subconscious belief system. The lie only demonstrates that the person is a liar...it is the effect.
- ❖ Except for love, the power of words inspired by a vision or fantasy is the most potent human force.

*For a dreamer: "Seeing is believing!"
*But they only see imaginary things that are not real!!
*This is why "The Secret" is WRONG!
*Say it and claim it is WRONG!
*Blab it and grab it IS WRONG!
*See it and be it IS WRONG!
Dreamers practice companionship – To be with someone or something!

VERY IMPORTANT:

1. Dreamers covet the object of their temptation, BUT they covet the temptation more so than the object itself because the temptation is the idol of their fantasy.
2. If there is a conflict between the conscious and subconscious mind, the subconscious mind always wins…ALWAYS!
3. All reaction occurs in the conscious mind; all interaction occurs in the subconscious mind. Fear is a "REACTION" to losing control.

For a visionary: "Believing is seeing!"

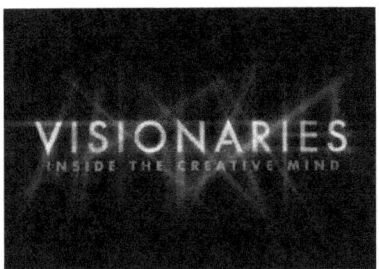

There are no SECRETS; there are only challenges to be conquered!

THIS IS NOT A SECRET: Putting a photo of a Ferrari on your refrigerator and seeing yourself driving it by employing the so-called law of attraction is pure BUPKES!!! Why? Because this is all occurring in the conscious mind and beliefs reside in the subconscious mind. How do you transfer something from the conscious mind to the subconscious mind and make it a belief system?

A Ferrari is the object of your temptation but what you covet most is the temptation of owning a Ferrari because the temptation is the idol of your fantasy.

It is all about ATTENTION & ACCEPTANCE!!!!! I have a $100 bill in my hand and I am willing to give it to you. But if you don't ACCEPT it then it is still in my hand. BELIEF SYSTEMS ARE CREATED BY ATTENTION & ACCEPTANCE!

John 1:12 But as many as received him, to them gave he **the right** to become children of God, *even* to them that believe on his name

Human things must be known to be loved; but divine things must be loved to be known.

BELIEVING IS SEEING!

Which of the following goals are good goals?

❖ To want to get married and have a wonderful, happy, loving marriage?
❖ To want to have children who are happy, successful, and loving?

- ❖ To have a successful, fulfilling and rewarding career?
- ❖ Is it a good goal to want to have fun, bonded, loving, and meaningful relationships with other people?

Which of the listed goals are good goals? None of them!

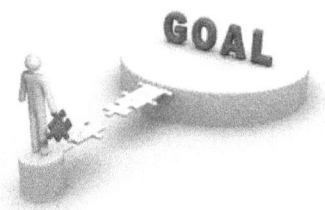

You should never have anything for a goal that is not 100% under your control, AND each and every goal should be <u>motivated by love</u>.

Almost all goals that we have in our life are wrong.

Everything that we do, we do because of a goal we have.

When we get up in the morning, it's because of some goal that we have; we are hungry for breakfast, or we need to go to work.

If we go to the grocery store, it's because of some goal we have. If we are kind to people, it's because of some goal that we have.

Now we don't always know what they are, because a lot of these are subconscious goals.

The goals we have are the reasons for everything we do. But, do all of your goals involve only YOU?

Of course not!

And when the other person, or persons, in your goal do not perform, or act the way you want them to, then we become anxious and stressed.

When our goals get blocked, it creates anger, anxiety, and frustration. If we only have good goals, we will not experience anger or anxiety.

That's how you know, if you are living a wrongful goal. If the result is anger and frustration because your control was blocked and blocking your goal, then you had a wrongful goal.

It may have been a fine and noble desire, but a wrongful goal.

Now, secular psychologists believe that the cause of illness is because of the way we **choose** to think or believe. Using cognitive therapy (Having a basis in or reducible to empirical factual knowledge.), they attempt to change a person's behavior and feelings.

But, we now know that illness is cured **not by changing our feelings or behavior,** but **by changing our beliefs and thoughts**. Does this sound like double-speak to you?

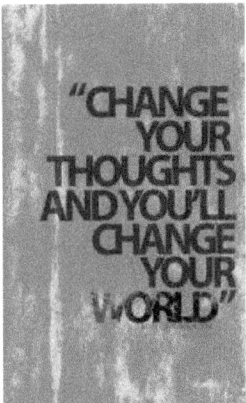

One of the things we will discuss is how men/women constantly confuse similar sounding terms, which have very separate and distinct meanings.

Perception and not reality rules human behavior! In the following, men/women commonly confuse:

- ❖ Faith vs. Hope
- ❖ Righteousness vs. Goodness
- ❖ Freedom vs. Liberty
- ❖ Rules vs. Ethics
- ❖ Quality vs. Quantity
- ❖ Quality of Life vs. Standard of Living
- ❖ Love vs. Lust
- ❖ Obligation vs. Legalism
- ❖ Wealth vs. Money
- ❖ Want vs. Need
- ❖ Machismo vs. Manhood
- ❖ Femininity vs. Womanhood
- ❖ War vs. Conflict
- ❖ Well-being vs. Being well
- ❖ Cause vs. Effect
- ❖ Relief vs. Cure
- ❖ Rationalization vs. Right
- ❖ Promise vs. Oath (Vow)
- ❖ Discipline vs. Punishment
- ❖ Taste vs. Substance
- ❖ Pain vs. Suffering
- ❖ Self-Control vs. Willpower

Okay…how does a person project themselves outward so that complete observation can occur?

Is it a matter of free will?

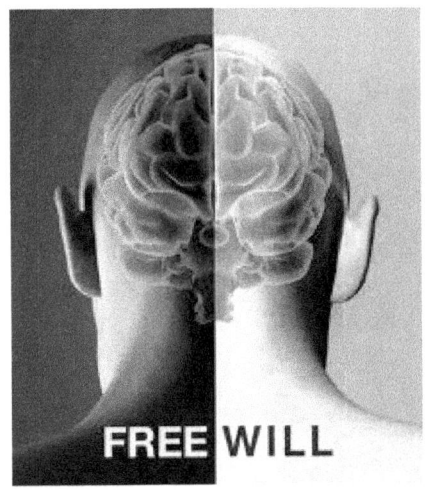

Let's talk about this for a moment and then there will be an exercise that begins teaching you this very attribute.

Chapter 3 – Free Will

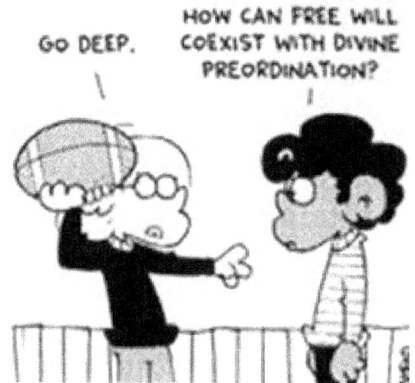

Much experimentation has occurred on the subject of free will. Does free will exist and does it act on the brain via attention?

I cite Ben Libet's now famous experiment in which subjects were asked to flex their wrists whenever they chose while being monitored by devices on their scalps, which were designed to measure the readiness potential, associated with preparation for movement. On average, the readiness potential was detected 550 milliseconds before movement occurred; however, not all readiness potentials were followed by movement. When subjects were asked to report when they were conscious of deciding to move, it was found that awareness preceded the movement by 100 to 200 milliseconds.

Some experts claim that this casts free will into doubt, as the signal to move came before awareness of the desire to move.

Libet posits that contrary to this disproving the existence of free will it is evidence that we are able to block the preparation process and stop movement from occurring altogether, since awareness still comes before movement.

Put this way it would seem as if <u>much of the will we exert is aimed to stop subconscious urges</u>, a concept called "free won't."

Libet believes that free will is not just the power to veto unbidden urges, though. He claims that free will is an active force.

Pointing to a plethora of experimental data, he says that willful mental effort is correlated with activity in the prefrontal cortex.

Repetitive (remember most learning is repetitive), automatic acts do not induce high amounts of activity in this area; whereas tasks involving concentration do (concentration or focus is a very important concept we will discuss more later on).

Schizophrenics show unusually low activity in this area, corresponding to lack of control.

Patients with lesions to the prefrontal cortex respond reflexively to environmental cues, performing actions with no thought.

From the experiments cited, it seems clear that this area of the brain is necessary for willful action, which Libet says in turn influences the brain.

What is all-important to this theory is attention.

Selective focusing of attention filters out distractions and makes one concentrate on one or a few particular elements present in sensory input. Although the data one receives is the same whether one is paying attention or not, the brain's response to the data is changed.

We can decide to some extent what information registers and what does not. Thus, our perceptions are changed. Or, to put it another way, mental force affects the activity of the brain in a perceptible way.

Given that we can change brain activity by paying attention to something, thus affecting the rate at which corresponding sets of synapses fire, it follows that attention is important for neuroplasticity (Neuroplasticity is the lifelong ability of the brain to reorganize neural pathways based on new experiences.

As we learn, we acquire new knowledge and skills through instruction or experience. In order to learn or memorize a fact or skill, there must be persistent functional changes in the brain that represent the new knowledge. The ability of the brain to change with learning is what is known as *neuroplasticity.*).

After all, as a certain neural pathway fires more and more often it becomes stronger and even more likely to be activated again. Just as sensory input can change cerebral cortex organization, PET scans have shown that attention can too (remember this fact because it is extremely important).

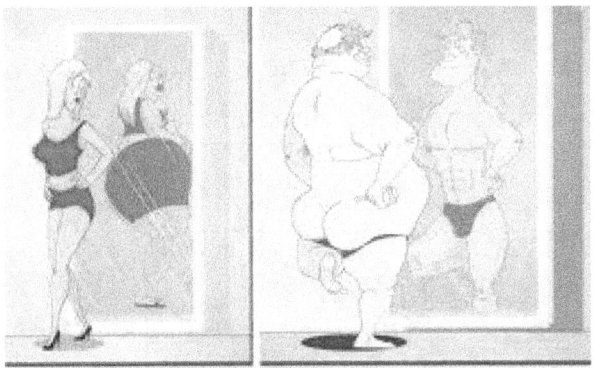

The Difference Between Women & Men
@FUGLY.COM

Libet even goes so far as to say that our mental states shape what we perceive more than the original stimulus does.

WOW! Did you understand this last comment? Our perceptions shape our responses and actions more than the reality or original stimuli!!! Reality versus perception rears its ugly head! Our mental state – the life force of focusing – shapes what we perceive more than the original stimulus.

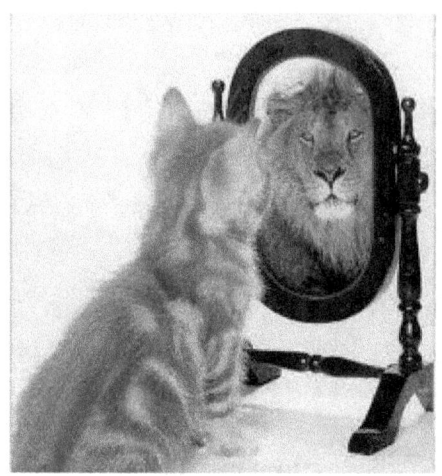

In other words, we are what we perceive and reality takes a back seat. We observe completely when our focus is away from ourselves.

This is very similar to "Zen" philosophy but more pure. Zen is about observation of "what is." Now, the 'what is' is the 'what is' *below* your filters and assumptions.

In other words, the goal and point of Zen is to watch your mind as it meaning-makes, while not attaching to either the process or your assumptions.

In this way, the mind sort of slides to the side, and you peer past the mind-games to the essential 'emptiness' of everything. (I don't believe this is true because Zen implies detachment and emptiness and I cannot abide either one of these. But what is certain, focusing your attention away from you will cause you to observe everything around you.)

Let's take our discussion a little bit farther for just a moment by discussing what is true or not true and how we arrive at truth.

I need you to see that your eyes and ears really do see and hear everything around you BUT, the mind deploys filters based on a variety of reasons that effectively block your awareness of the various stimuli.

Chapter 4 – The Incredible Power of Focus

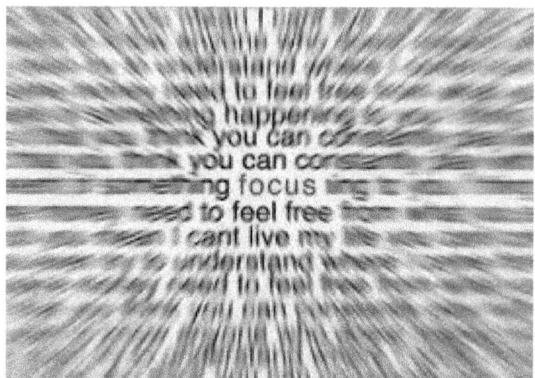

One important point to make is the idea that you really do create your own life and your own reality. Many people, after continuing to experience the same old ups and downs and personal dramas over many years, get to the point where they dismiss this idea as charming but useless -- or just plain wrong.

"If I'm creating this, then I'm certainly not doing it on purpose," they say. "It sure seems like this is HAPPENING to me, rather than that I'm creating it."

They just assume that it's all BS because "this and this and this and this are going on for me, and I have no control over it, and anyone who thinks I'm creating this doesn't understand what I'm going through."

Essentially, they are resigning themselves to becoming a victim of circumstances... the Central You!

We live in a universe of infinite complexity and many forces that operate on us -- way too many to keep track of.

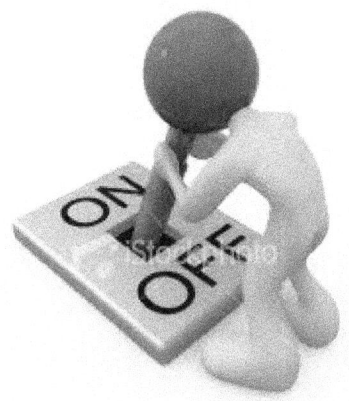

Yes, it is true that we are NOT in control of everything that happens because we are not in control of most of those infinite other parts of the universe.

In fact, the only thing you have total and complete control over is YOUR OWN MIND; that is, if you learn how to exercise it.

Control over your mind gives you tremendous power. By exercising control over your mind, you can get the rest of those infinite other parts of the universe to begin to march in formation.

The person who says, "If I'm creating this, it certainly isn't on purpose," is right. They are not creating what is happening to them "on purpose."

Who would purposely create failure, or bad relationships, or any other kind of suffering? You can only do something that is not good for you - that is harmful to you - if you do it <u>subconsciously</u>.

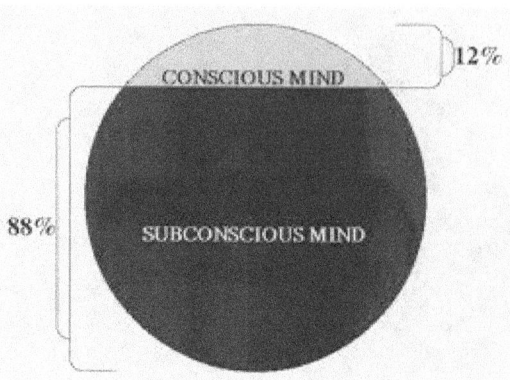

This means if you are creating something you don't want, you must be doing so subconsciously. Your mind is running on automatic pilot, based on the "software" (subconscious programming) installed when you were too young to know any better, by parents, teachers, friends, the media, and other experiences and influences.

The key is to become more conscious, more aware...to get yourself off automatic pilot. Once you do this, you stop creating all the dramas and other garbage you don't want in your life.

How do you do this? One way is by remembering and using a very important piece of wisdom. What is this important piece of wisdom? I'm glad you asked...

Whatever you focus on manifests as reality in your life
You are always focusing on something, whether you are aware of it or not. If I spent some time with you, and heard your history, I could tell you what you are focusing on. How? By looking at the results you are getting in your life.

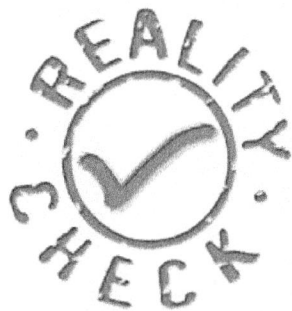

The results are always the result of your focus. The problem is this focus is usually not conscious focus; it's automatic or subconscious focus. We subconsciously focus on something we don't want, and then when we get it we feel like a victim and don't even stop to think that we created it in the first place.

We don't realize we could choose to create something completely different if we could only get out of the cycle of subconsciously focusing on something other than what we want.

Focusing on what you do not want, ironically, makes it happen.

Focusing on not being poor makes you poor.

Focusing on not making mistakes causes you to make mistakes.

Focusing on not having a bad relationship creates bad relationships.

Focusing on not being depressed makes you depressed.

Focusing on not smoking makes you want to smoke.

And so on. I think you get the idea. The mind will create what you focus on both GOOD and BAD!!!

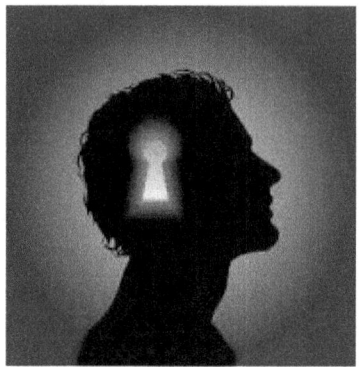

Focusing the Mind

The truth is your mind cannot tell the difference between something you think about or focus on that you DO want, and something you think about or focus on but do NOT want.

The mind is a goal-seeking mechanism, and an extremely effective one at that. Already, all the time, it is elegantly and precisely creating exactly what you focus on. You are already a World Champion Expert at creating whatever you focus on. You couldn't get any better at it, and you don't need to get any better at it.

When you focus on anything, your mind says: "Okay, we can do that," and starts figuring out how to do it.

It doesn't ask whether you're focusing on it because you want it or because you do not want it. It ALWAYS assumes you want what you focus on and then it goes and makes it happen.

The more frequent and the more intense the focus, the faster and more completely you will create what you have focused on, which is why intense negative experiences create intense focus on what you do not want, and tend to make you re-create what you don't want, over and over.

Conscious Intention

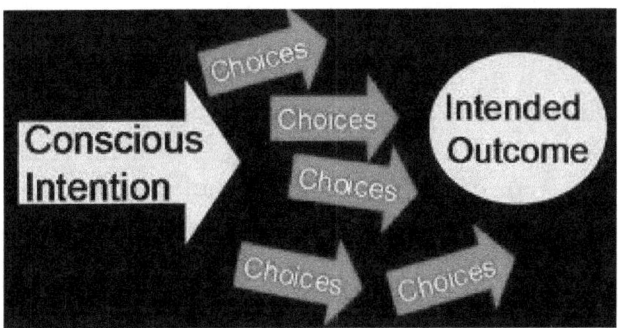

Most of the time, for most people, all the focusing and thinking is going by at warp speed, on automatic, without much, if any, conscious intention. Our job today is to learn how to direct this power by consciously directing your focus to the outcomes you want. Once you do, everything changes.

This does, however, take some work, because at first you have to swim upstream against the current of your old, unconscious habits, and the current can be swift and strong. Trained observation actually teaches you to focus on what you want.

First, you have to discover all the things you focus on that you do not want, and I'm willing to bet there are quite a few -- way more than you think.

To the degree you're getting what you don't want, you are focusing, albeit subconsciously, on what you don't want.

Spend some time over the next few weeks making a list of all the things you do NOT want as you notice yourself thinking about them.

Second, you have to get very clear about what you DO want.

Then, you have to examine each of the things you want and be sure they are not just something you do NOT want in disguise. For instance, saying "I want a relationship where I am treated well" would not even be an issue if you had not had relationships where you were not treated well, and even in making this seemingly positive statement you are focusing on not wanting to be mistreated.

Saying "I want a reliable car" wouldn't even come up if you weren't focusing on the fact that you don't want a car that breaks down and needs a lot of repairs.

After you've sorted out the things you habitually focus on that you do not want, and know what you do want, you have to begin to notice each time you think about an outcome you do not want, and consciously change your thinking, right in that moment, so you're instead focusing on what you do want.

Remember, you do NOT have to avoid things to be happy and get what you want. The urge to avoid something is a result of having had a negative emotional experience regarding that thing, and trying to avoid things requires you to focus on them, which tells your brain to create them. Not good.

You will be surprised how often you are thinking about what you do not want, how difficult it is to catch yourself doing it every time, and -- most of all – how difficult it is to switch your thinking to what you DO want.

The solution?

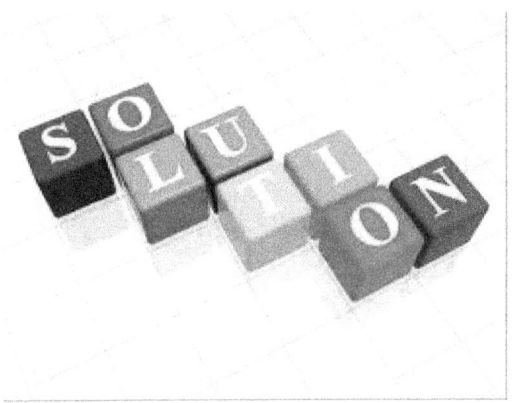

Practice, practice, practice! Persistence, persistence, persistence!!! It's a very good idea to write down what you want, very specifically, so that your Fairy Godmother, were she to read it, would know exactly what to give you without any additional explanation. Then, read what you have written to yourself, preferably out loud, several times a day, while seeing yourself, in your mind, already having what you want.

Believing is seeing and not the other way around as the world teaches you!

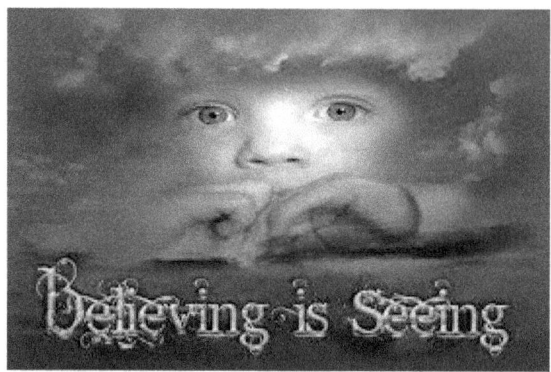

Another way to change your focus is to ask questions. As an example, I'll ask you one right now. What did you have for breakfast this morning? To answer this question (even to just internally process the question), you had to shift your focus from whatever your mind was focused on (hopefully, to what I am teaching) to today's breakfast. This means that to change your focus, all you have to do is...ask yourself a question!

Chapter 5 – 3-Steps to Controlling Your Mind

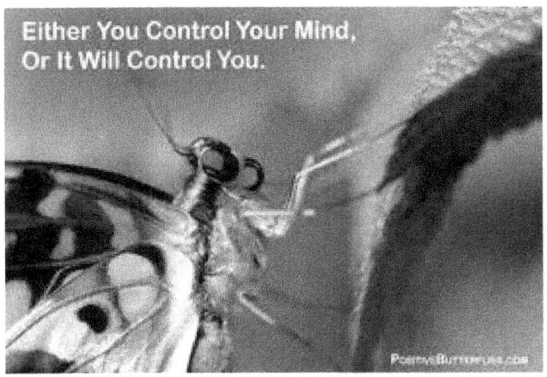

1. Awareness

The first step to changing anything is becoming aware that it's happening, especially if it's your mind.

Pretend your mind is racing, and you finally realize that you're thinking. Most people at this stage get extremely frustrated and "try" to force their mind into submission.

It doesn't work! Why? Because, what you focus on expands. The more frustrated you get, the more you're focusing on frustration, so you'll get even MORE frustration and more thinking... on and on!

So the first step is to simply become "aware" of the fact that you're thinking.

Nothing more! When you notice that you're thinking, smile to yourself, and say, "I just noticed myself thinking... interesting..."

Now notice what happens inside of you when you do this... something VERY profound. If "I" just noticed "myself" thinking, perhaps there are really two completely separate identities running your life? There is the "I" and there is the "self."

The Power of Choice

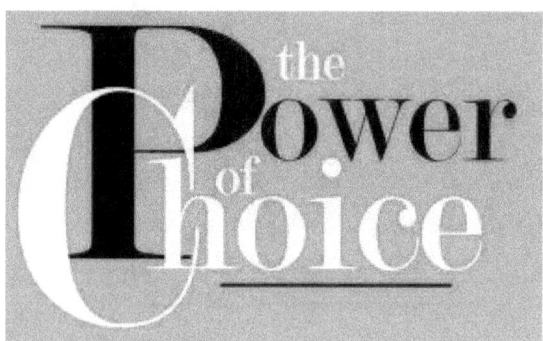

The "I", is the real you...the intellect, the "I" behind the mind, that runs the show, the heart, the soul, the true conscious being, the choice maker.

The "self" is the desires, emotions and will of the mind; if left to run the show, it will run in endless circles until the edge of insanity.

The moment you do this, the moment you become "aware" - you are no longer a slave to your mind. You have won.

After you become aware... do nothing, just lay there for 3 seconds and notice how it feels to be present in who you really are, not the mind, but you, the "I" - there is a great feeling of peace behind that presence in the "I." Why?

Because when you are aware like this, you're aware of the power of your choice making. You now have the power of choice.

2. Relaxed Focus

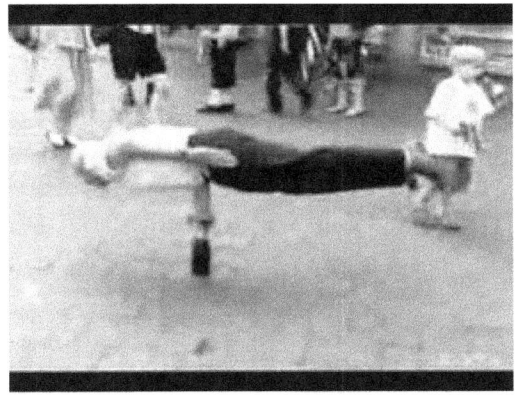

"What you focus on expands."

Now that you have become aware of your thinking, all you have to do is "direct" your mind into a place that will bring you into a deep, deep place of relaxation.

Think about it, if before your mind will relentlessly race into any direction you give it; why not pick a direction that will give you peace and restful sleep?

But, most people don't know what that direction really is. It's really easy. If you focus on anything your body does or feels subconsciously, you will begin to become more and more relaxed.

For example your breathing, the feeling of the pillow on your head, the sounds of nature outside (unless you live in the city), the warmth of your body.

These are all things that happen, yet your conscious mind doesn't think about them. As you know, "What you focus on expands"... So what would happen if you focused on something that is happening in your "subconscious"?

That's right, your conscious thinking would diminish, and your subconscious mind would begin to take over the entire process of you falling asleep!

It really is that simple, and it works every time. The easiest one is your breathing. And I promise you if you just try this tonight, you will be shocked: "Wow! It worked!"

3. Repetition

Repetition
Repetition
Repetition

As I said, the easiest one to focus on is your breathing. In the beginning, you'll find this easier said than done. Begin by taking your focus onto your breathing.

Take a deep breath in; hold it for a short while, slowly exhale.

Count "1" Breathe in again; hold it shortly, exhale slowly, and count..."2". Why count?

Because in the very beginning, you may find it challenging to hold your focus. In fact, you'll be surprised as you may not even make it to "5" the first time.

This is because your subconscious ever-thinking mind will butt in and interrupt.

You may randomly go off into a barrage of thoughts again. If this happens, what do you do? Simply become aware, and begin focusing on your breathing again.

As you become aware, 2 or 3 times, your mind will give up. When you get to "10" or "15" breaths you will feel a wave of relaxation in your body. This is the silent "click" as your mind shifts from the high frequency Beta brain-waves into Alpha brain-waves.

Your subconscious mind will do the rest! The following exercise will teach you how to see and recognize things that are unworthy of attention, but still recognize that they are there.

In other words, attention will be paid to it and then discarded CONSCIOUSLY.

EXERCISE #1

You look but you do not see: First of all, I want you to get a pencil and paper and find a painting in your home.

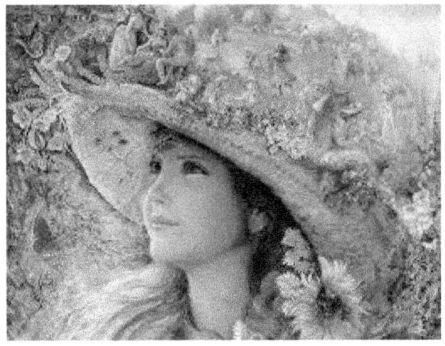

Place a chair in front of the painting and write down everything you see. Do not stop until you have listed at least 100 aspects of the painting.

Be sure to look at every aspect of the painting. Project yourself outside of your subconscious mind. This exercise is designed to keep you in your conscious mind for observation purposes.

The way you perceive the painting is different than seeing the painting. Seeing the painting is first, perception is second. Do you see the difference?

No one is asking you to tell us how you feel, just recognize what is in the painting.

Feelings are from the subconscious mind; reality is conscious. Stick with reality when you see.

A women will list the emotional aspects of the painting such as, "the colors are warm" or maybe, "the women are dressed nicely and trying to impress the men."

Here you will begin to see that you are allowing emotions to take over. Look physically at the painting. Yes, note the colors but not how they make you feel.

Men have a tendency to list the physical aspects such as, "It takes place in this big field" or maybe, "The picture is rectangular and in a very ugly frame."

Men have it easier in this exercise than women because men employ their psyches in the physical and intellectual planes. Women employ their psyches on an emotional and spiritual plane.

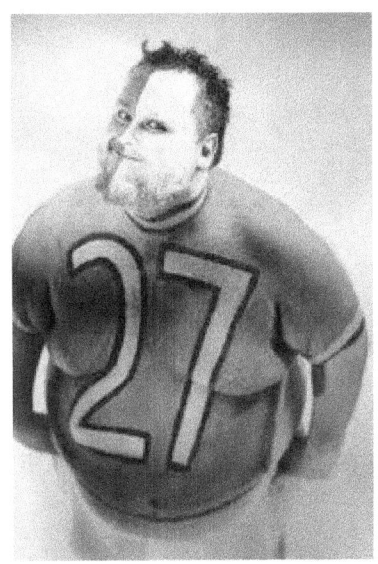

In this exercise I want both men and women to list only their physical observations. It doesn't matter which painting you use; writing down 100 aspects is pretty simple once you get the hang of it.

THINK outside the envelope of emotions. Look and observe and try to see what is there.

If you continue to do this often, with different paintings, you will find that wherever you go you will begin to pick out details that eluded you in the past WITH NO EMOTIONAL BAGGAGE ATTACHED.

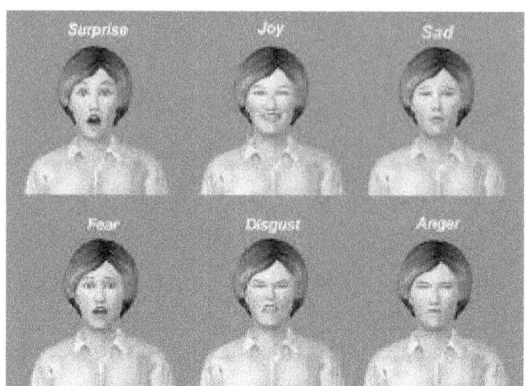

Pretty soon, with some good effort, you will begin to look at pictures as a snapshot in your mind and pick out all of the details

Let's talk about the pictures of the heart. These pictures are your belief system. We animate these pictures into either fantasies or visions.

A newborn baby, suffering from neglect from its mother, does not have language to express his/her anguish. Even when it develops language and ages, the baby cannot consciously remember the neglect, but the pictures stored in his/her subconscious are still there and manifest themselves by affecting the thought process.

After the thought process I have described, we express these fantasies, or visions, through action, which in turn, is called behavior and conduct.

Past experience plays a very major part in present behavior/conduct, but not all childhood traumas translates into adult behavior.

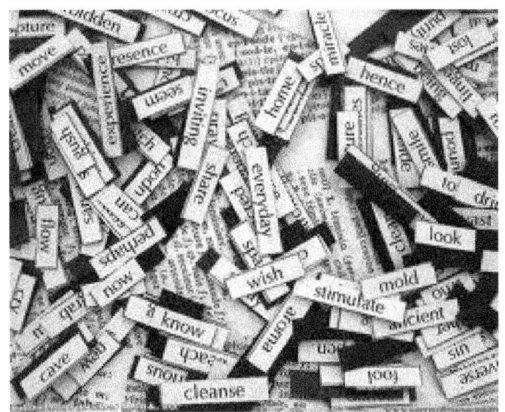

Another such action is words! Except for love, the power of words, inspired by a vision, or fantasy, is the most potent human force. Visions evoke strength; fantasies evoke power, and there is a very big difference between strength and power.

Visions are good; most fantasies are bad, but a healthy fantasy is not to be discarded. The mind works by the ear! Words create pictures and pictures talk back. The inner dialogue is called thinking.

Sub-conscience thinking is the combining of sounds and perceived images. How a person feels about this unconscious dialogue, determines "conscious decisions."

If we don't feel anything, our hearts say, in effect, "Return to sender." We constantly want to feel and demonstrate these feelings. This is the inherent problem between love and lust.

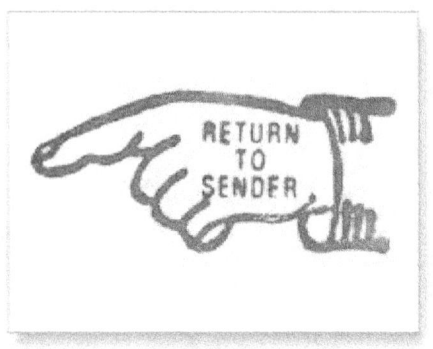

Love is born in the intellect and seeks communion. Lust is born in the emotions and seeks companionship."

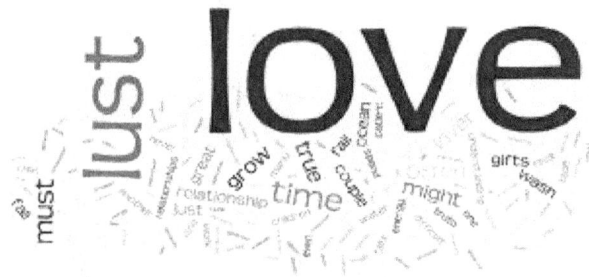

What we see, we then animate into pictures, and the mind stores these images, and forms its belief systems from them. If you don't SEE all of the details you only have a partial picture.

Imagine seeing an ocean without waves, or flowers without color? Partial pictures form wrongful belief systems. All "seeing" eventually makes it into the subconscious mind because the human mind chooses to react to all stimuli entering the five senses.

However; to avoid filters you must train the mind to pay attention to what is seen FIRST in the conscious mind and then the subconscious mind takes over.

Let's go one step further. What you are doing with this exercise is teaching your subconscious mind that every detail is important AFTER the conscious mind pays attention to it FIRST.

In the past, you looked at something and your mind only remembered what your subconscious mind thought was important; however, now you are REPETITIVELY teaching it that everything is important CONSCIOUSLY FIRST.

This is how the mind learns, and this is why your teachers always assigned homework and you had to repetitively cram for finals. The mind learns by repetition – CONSCIOUS AND SUBCONSCIOUS!

Now it makes a man wonder, can this be the answer to all of your problems? What if you can train the mind in the opposite direction…REPETITIVELY!

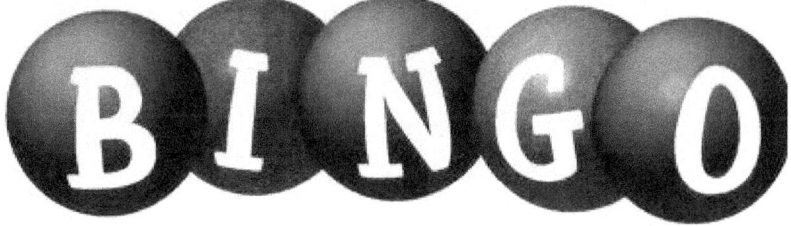

BINGO, this is exactly what we behavioral scientists do, in order to get you away from wrongful behavior.

Remember the mind uses the very same mechanism to learn good things as well as bad things. It is just that you have perceived that bad things are more fun.

And seeing bad things can really be more fun. Happiness and pleasure, in the short-term, seems to outweigh long-term joy!

Listen up: short-term happiness has a tendency to push away long-term joy, so be aware of this and strive for the long-term joy. It is simply a matter of training yourself to do it!

Chapter 6 – More on Focusing

The one thing in your life you can command is your own mind. Whatever negative people and situations you face, you can always choose a positive attitude. But doing so requires a firm, strong commitment.

Helpful: Begin by writing a self-convincing creed – I believe I can direct and control my emotions, intellect and habits with the intention of developing a positive mental attitude.

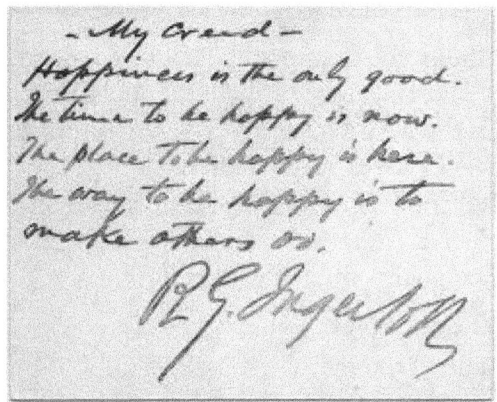

Post it where you'll see it when you get up in the morning. Read it during the day, and say it aloud. Speaking an intention reinforces it.

Choose a "self-motivator" – a meaningful phrase tailored to help you reach your positive thinking goals. Examples:

❖ Counter discouragement with the phrase "Every problem contains the seed of its own solution."

❖ Fight procrastination with "Do it now."

Keep your self-motivators nearby – in your pocket or on your desk – and repeat them throughout the day to instill these important new values.

Develop a Life Plan

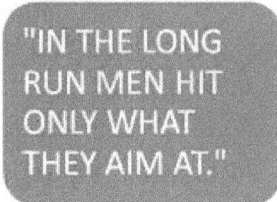

"IN THE LONG RUN MEN HIT ONLY WHAT THEY AIM AT."

• HENRY DAVID THOREAU

Setting short and long-term goals each day creates a road map for your life. But only set GOOD goals!!! What is a good goal? One where you are 100% in control and one that is founded in love! A goal of raising good, healthy and prosperous children is a bad goal because you are not in control of what your kids choose. See the important difference? The goal is noble but it is not a good goal.

You identify where you're going, focus your mind on getting there and avoid many wrong turns.

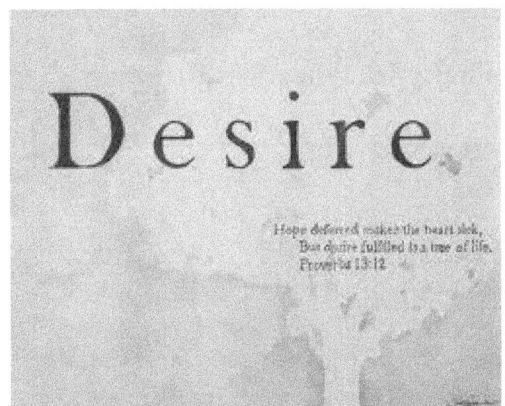

Desire

Hope deferred makes the heart sick,
But desire fulfilled is a tree of life.
Proverbs 13:12

Helpful: Use the D-E-S-I-R-E formula as a goal-setting guideline...

❖ **D**etermine what you want. Be exact, and express the goal positively. Say what you want to be or do rather than what you don't want.

❖ **E**valuate what you'll give in return. How much work will you do to turn your plan into action?

❖ **S**et a date for your goal. Be realistic, allowing enough time without postponing it too long.

❖ **I**dentify a step by step plan. Devise immediate, small steps to get started.

❖ **R**epeat your plan in writing.

❖ **E**ach and every day, morning and evening, read your plan aloud as you picture yourself already having achieved your goals.

Writing out your daily goals helps maintain your motivation.

Keep them in your pocket or purse to read frequently throughout the day.

Chapter 7 - PhattyFat Wheytloss Diet Plan

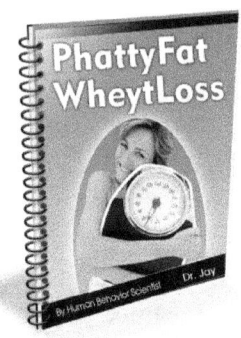

Here is a simple diet program I use to maintain my optimum weight level. Contrary to what some knuckleheads claim, this is not a starvation diet. The body burns the most calories when digesting protein so even if you use another diet program, always drink a protein shake before going to bed.

A few things to note: Do not eat any carbs at any time with this program otherwise the presence of glucose (sugar) will negate the protein intake.

Furthermore, do not stay on this diet more than six weeks.

What you will need:

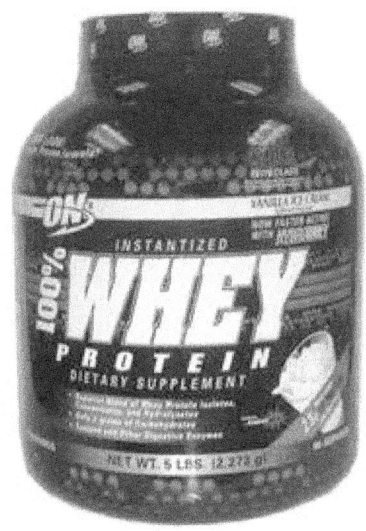

1st 10-days:

Whey Protein Powder for shakes – you want "whey protein" and nothing else. The best quality is at GNC Nutrition Stores but it is expensive ($45-$60 depending on when you buy it; they offer sales at the beginning of each month).

If budget is a consideration Walmart offers a product called, "Body Fortress" Super Advanced Whey Protein. It costs under $15 and it works.

I use it because I am basically "cheap" but it's your call. It comes in three flavors – chocolate, strawberry and vanilla. I prefer the chocolate but it is your call again.

Shaker Cup – buy it at Walmart; it costs $1.25.

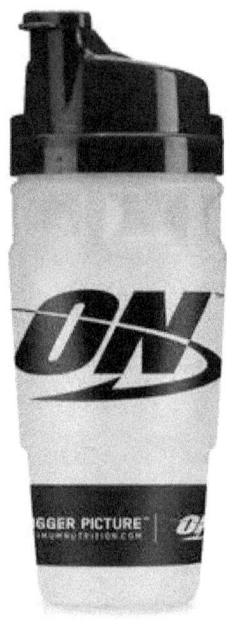

After 10-days to 3 or 4-weeks

Turkey Breast – any high quality turnkey breast will do EXCEPT lunch meat. This contains way too much salt.

Note: Do not cut corners. Follow my instructions to a tee. I have trained professional actors, professional models and literally thousands of people on this program. It works IF you allow it to work! And if you have learned anything from this book, it is all about denial of self and focusing on a weight loss condition. YOU MUST LEASRN SELF DENIAL AND WHEN YOU DO LIFE WILL BE GRAND!

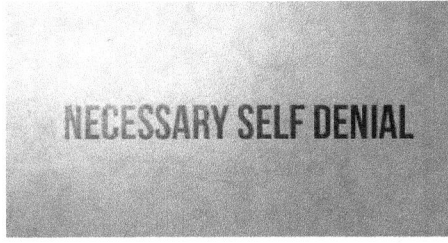

NECESSARY SELF DENIAL

1st 10-days

Drink a shake every 4-hours and right before bedtime too! No forget right before bedtime!! Remember, the body's preferred fuel source is FAT, then protein and then sugar.

It takes the least amount of calories to burn sugar and the most to burn fat. Protein sits right in the middle. You lose weight because the body requires the calories you have stored as fat to digest the protein.

The first two days is the toughest as you body will signal that it is hungry and the fact that more than likely you are addicted to carbs.

After the first couple of days these hunger pangs will go away. Beginning about the third day the weight will begin to come off.

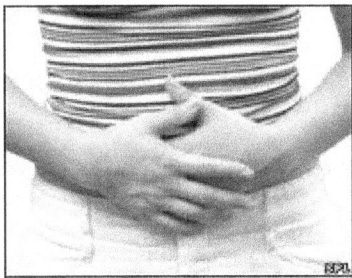

Weigh yourself every morning because as you see the weight loss you become more committed.

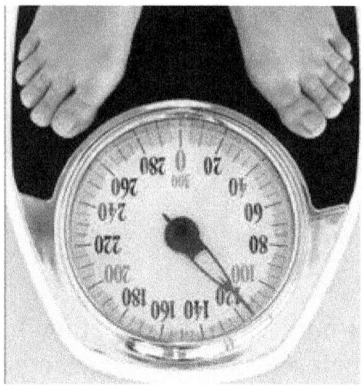

Follow this program for 10-days. After 10-days you need to begin to gradually eat again beginning with the turkey breast described above.

You can eat about 6 0zs of turkey breast, 4-times/day. I spruce up my meal with sliced jalapenos or peppercinis.

You can even have some vegetables but not a lot. You need to gradually get back into eating. You do this from 10-days up to 3-4 weeks.

After 3-4 weeks (depending if you have reached your weight loss goals) you can once again begin eating regular meals but...BUT...if you go back to your previous habits SHAME ON YOU!!! Then you have not learned anything!

Eat in moderation and then you can eat anything you want.

In a three week periods of time the average weight loss 16-18 lbs. Yeah, it works.

NOTE: THIS PROGRAM IS NOT A REGULAR MENU PLAN. DO NOT STAY ON A PROTEIN DIET. AFTER 4-WEEKS MAXIMUM GET OFF OF

Exercise

You need to exercise. I am 60-years old so I walk twice a day for about 3 or 4-miles. It is relaxing and I meet some interesting people. It also allows me to walk my dog and I know he loves it.

You can do strenuous exercising but select an exercise program that you can commit to and keep up with over the long term.

That's it! It is simple and it works. Best of luck!

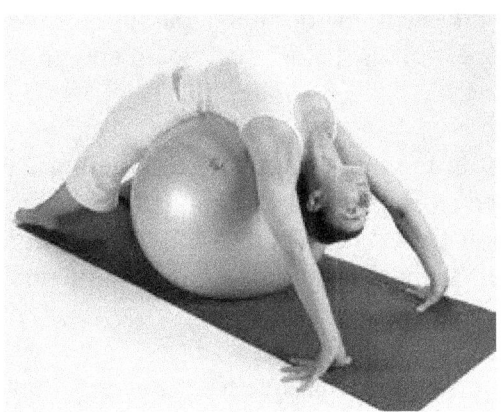

I Have a Special Gift for My Readers

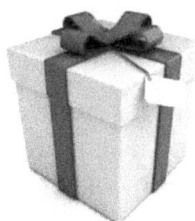

I appreciate my readers for without them I am just another author attempting to make a difference. If my book has made a favorable impression please leave me an honest review. Thank you in advance for you participation.

My readers and I have in common a passion for the written word as well as the desire to learn and grow from books.

My special offer to you is a massive ebook library that I have compiled over the years. It contains hundreds of fiction and non-fiction ebooks in Adobe Acrobat PDF format as well as the Greek classics and old literary classics too.

In fact, this library is so massive to completely download the entire library will require over 5 GBs open on your desktop.

Use the link below and scan all of the ebooks in the library. You can select the ebooks you want individually or download the entire library.

The link below does not expire after a given time period so you are free to return for more books rather than clog your desktop. And feel free to give the link to your friends who enjoy reading too.

I thank you for reading my book and hope if you are pleased that you will leave me an honest review so that I can improve my work and or write books that appeal to your interests.

Okay, here is the link…

http://tinyurl.com/special-readers-promo

PS: If you wish to reach me personally for any reason you may simply write to mailto:support@epubwealth.com.

I answer all of my emails so rest assured I will respond.

Meet the Author

Dr. Harry Jay is Director of Research for AppliedMindSciences.com, a mental health and mind research group of Applied Web Info, and is the author of over 100 books and research papers as a behavioral scientist.

In his 32-year career, Dr. Harry Jay has contributed many new mental health treatment treatments and protocols using some of the new advances he has discovered in Energy Psychology.

He specializes in addictions of all kinds, sexual abuse, child predation and gender relationships.

He is also a board member to ePubWealth.com and serves on the science committee assisting non-fiction science writers in book publishing and promotion.

As a leading behavioral scientist, he provides profiling services to the company's ForensicsNation.com unit as well as criminal psychology research to aid in identifying and apprehending child predators and cyber-criminals of all kinds.

He resides in Southern Utah and enjoys the outdoors, fishing and photography.

Visit some of his websites
http://www.AddMeInNow.com
http://www.AppliedMindSciences.com

http://www.AppliedWebInfo.com
http://www.BookbuilderPLUS.com
http://www.BookJumping.com
http://www.EmailNations.com
http://www.EmbarrassingProblemsFix.com
http://www.ePubWealth.com
http://www.ForensicsNation.com
http://www.ForensicsNationStore.com
http://www.FreebiesNation.com
http://www.HealthFitnessWellnessNation.com
http://www.Neternatives.com
http://www.PrivacyNations.com
http://www.RetireWithoutMoney.org
http://www.SurvivalNations.com
http://www.TheBentonKitchen.com
http://www.Theolegions.org
http://www.VideoBookbuilder.com